ARYA SKYE

THE SKINCARE LAB

Crafting your unique formula for skin success

First edition

This book was professionally typeset on Reedsy.
Find out more at reedsy.com

Your skin is your canvas upon which your
stories unfold

Arya Skye

Contents

1

Introduction

Welcome to The Skincare Lab, a comprehensive guide to understanding, optimizing, and mastering the art of skincare. In this chapter, we will explore the purpose of this book, take an overview of skincare, delve into our unique approach, and discuss the comprehensive insights and practical applications it offers.

The purpose of The Skincare Lab is to provide you with a holistic understanding of skincare that goes beyond mere product recommendations. Our goal is to empower you with knowledge, enabling you to make informed decisions about your skincare routine, products, and lifestyle choices.

Skincare is a multifaceted and dynamic field, encompassing a wide range of topics, including the structure and function of the skin, common skin concerns, aging, environmental impacts, and more. In the coming chapters, we will provide an in-depth overview of these essential aspects, ensuring that you have a solid foundation on which to build your skincare knowledge.

Our approach to skincare is unique in that we emphasize a personalized, well-rounded approach. We believe that effective skincare goes beyond external treatments and requires an understanding of internal factors such as nutrition, hormones, gut health, stress management, and lifestyle. By addressing skincare from a holistic perspective, we aim to equip you with the tools to nurture your skin from the inside out.

Within these pages, you will find comprehensive insights that bridge the gap between scientific knowledge and practical application. We will explore the latest research, ingredient science, and skincare trends, presenting them in an accessible and engaging manner, so you can make the best choices for your skin.

Moreover, practical applications and tools will be a core focus of The Skincare Lab. From creating personalized skincare routines to understanding how to select products and ingredients tailored to your needs, we will provide you with actionable steps and tools that you can integrate seamlessly into your daily skincare regimen.

So, come with us on this journey as we explore the world of skincare, gain comprehensive insights, and acquire practical applications to elevate your skincare routine from ordinary to extraordinary. Welcome to The Skincare Lab.

2

A Crash Course into Skin

The skin, the largest organ of the human body, serves as the ultimate barrier and the most profound canvas of individual appearance. Marvelously complex, it works tirelessly to protect against external harm while maintaining a delicate internal balance. This chapter delves into the intricacies of our skin, acknowledging its vital functions, examining the factors that influence its health, distinguishing between different skin types, considering the particular needs of skin of color, and emphasizing the importance of skincare knowledge for overall well-being.

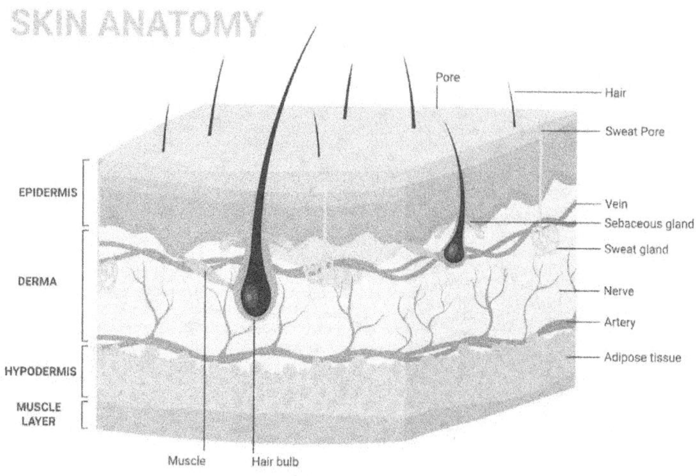

Skin Anatomical Overview

To fully grasp skincare, one must first understand the structure of the skin. The skin is composed of three primary layers:

The Epidermis: The outermost barrier that shields the body against environmental threats and prevents moisture loss. It is where we find skin cells, pigment, and proteins.

The Dermis: Directly beneath the epidermis, fortified with collagen and elastin fibers, it houses nerve endings, glands, and follicles. It provides strength and elasticity.

The Hypodermis: This deeper layer contains fat and connective tissue and functions as insulation and cushioning for the body.

A thorough understanding of these layers and their specific roles lays the groundwork for grasping how skincare products and treatments interact with our skin.

Skin Functions

The functions of the skin are vital and multifaceted. It protects internal tissues from mechanical impacts, pathogens, and the elements. Skin plays a central role in thermoregulation, immune defense, and sensory perception. It also synthesizes Vitamin D when exposed to sunlight, which is essential for bone health. Recognizing these functions is pivotal for appreciating why skincare is not merely cosmetic, but also a health imperative.

Factors Influencing Skin Health

Several factors influence skin health:

Environmental Factors: Sun exposure, pollution, and weather conditions can cause damage or premature aging.

Lifestyle Choices: Diet, sleep patterns, and stress levels influence skin's appearance and resilience.

Genetic Makeup: Genetic predispositions can determine skin sensitivity and propensity for certain skin conditions.

Hormonal Changes: Fluctuations, especially during puberty, pregnancy, or menopause, impact skin behavior.

Age: Aging naturally changes skin's structure and function.

Understanding these factors can help tailor skincare routines more effectively.

Identifying Skin Types

A cornerstone of skincare is identifying one's skin type, generally categorized as:

Normal: Balanced oil and moisture levels.
Dry: Flaky, itchy, or rough due to insufficient sebum.
Oily: Shiny and prone to acne due to excess sebum.
Combination: Oily in some areas (like the T-zone) and dry in others.
Sensitive: Prone to inflammation and irritation.
Recognizing which type one's skin aligns with can guide the selection of appropriate products and routines.

Skin Color

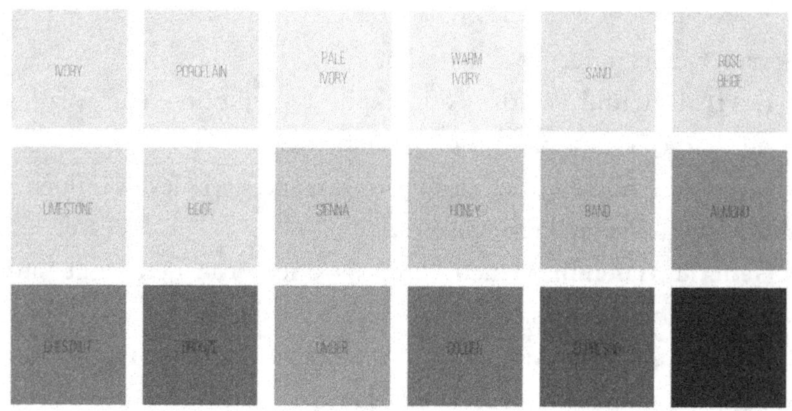

Skin color has unique characteristics and concerns, such as hyper-pigmentation and keloid formation. Recognizing these differences is crucial for proper skin care. Moreover, products and treatments must address the distinct needs of melanin-rich skin, avoiding one-size-fits-all approaches to skincare.

Importance of Skincare Knowledge

Illuminating the why's and how's of caring for one's skin equips individuals with the power to make informed decisions, avoid common pitfalls, and proactively address issues. Skincare knowledge is not superficial—it is an investment in one's health and self-esteem.

When armed with comprehensive understanding, individuals can craft a skincare routine that respects the skin's complexity and honors its role as a life-sustaining and identity-defining organ.

Our skin is an extraordinary organ, deserving of recognition and care. This crash course into its layers, functions, and the nuances of its care serves as a foundation towards a more refined and educated approach to skincare. With every cream applied and routine followed, it's a step towards health, confidence, and radiance.

3

The Vital Canvas: The Importance of Taking Care of Your Skin

In the grand tapestry of our body's organs, the skin asserts a unique presence, an interface between our inner machinations and the world beyond. This chapter delves into the profound significance of diligent skincare as a practice not merely cosmetic, but holistic in ensuring overall well-being, shielding against environmental onslaughts, mirroring our systemic health, decelerating the sands of time, and nurturing our psychological tranquility.

Overall Well-Being

Vigor, vitality, and health are inextricably linked with our outermost layer. Skin, the body's largest organ, performs miraculous functions— from regulating body temperature to synthesizing vital Vitamin D. Skincare, thus, transcends aesthetic appeal; it is self-care. A routine as simple as moisturizing can fortify the skin's barrier, preventing the ingress of pathogens, and maintaining hydration balance, which is pivotal for cellular health and preventive against systemic diseases that might arise from cracked or compromised skin.

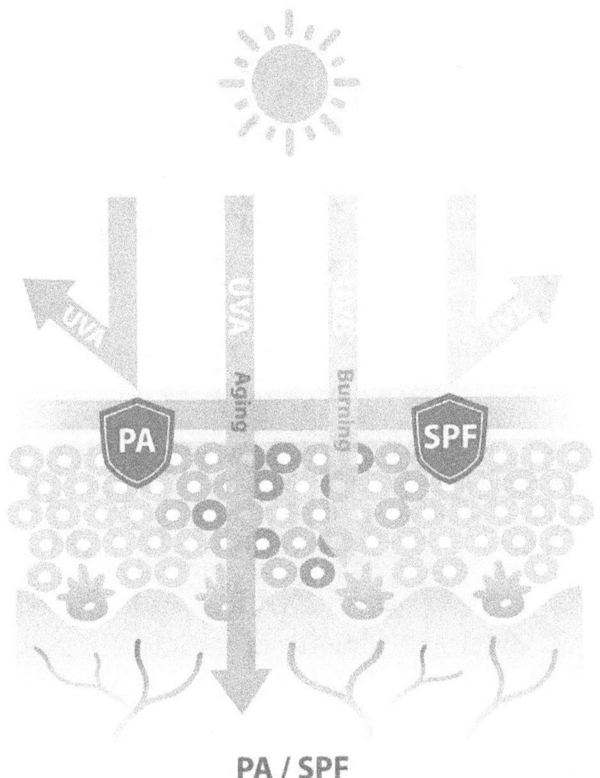

Protection from Environmental Factors

Our skin is constantly besieged by environmental villains—UV rays, pollution, smoke, and so forth. Left unguarded, the skin bears the brunt, sustaining damage at a cellular level. Herein lies your essence of sunscreens, antioxidants, and cleansing rituals. These guardians of the epidermis help in repelling these assaults, reducing the risk of skin cancers and preserving the integrity of skin cells. Protective skincare forms the first line of defense against a world rife with invisible adversaries.

Skin as a Reflection of Health

Peering into the mirror, the reflection one beholds is more than skin-deep. It is a narrative of one's internal health. Conditions like dehydration manifest as dry patches, while allergies and nutritional deficits declare their presence through rashes and breakouts. Thus, skincare is a form of dialogue with our bodies, where maintaining a radiant, healthy complexion often stems from a balanced diet, adequate hydration, and attuned living habits.

Preventing Premature Aging

Chronology cannot be outpaced, yet with meticulous skincare, one can slow the unwelcome advance of premature aging. Factors such as repeated sun exposure, smoking, and repetitive facial expressions etch lines into our stories far earlier than we might wish. A regimen composed of retinoids, peptides, and hydration works not only to pacify the present but to invest in a time-defiant future. Consequently, preventive skincare is less about vanquishing the inevitable and more about cherishing the age you are at every stage of life.

Psychological Benefits

Lastly, the act of skincare is intrinsically therapeutic, a ritual where one tends to the self with intention and care. This tactile engagement is a form of mindfulness, soothing for the mind as much as it is for the skin. Furthermore, self-perception is intimately tied to skin health. The confidence that emanates from clear, healthy skin is seen not only in the radiance of one's visage but in the assertive stride of their steps.

Healthy skin contributes to a positive self-image and bolsters mental well-being.

As we draw this chapter to a close, it's clear that skincare is a profound compass in the journey of self-care. It is our armor in the battle against the elements, a revealing map of our well-being, a chronicle of our life's tales, and an origin of psychological solace. To prioritize skincare is to honor the very vehicle that will carry us through a lifetime of experiences. Thus, let us wield this knowledge as we would the finest cream, anointing ourselves with the precepts of comprehensive self-care. Our skin is not just an organ; it is the canvas upon which our life stories are etched, and it warrants our utmost reverence and care.

4

Basic Skincare

In the journey to maintain healthy, vibrant skin, understanding the fundamentals of skincare is an essential stepping stone. From the dewy youthfulness of a child's complexion to the seasoned skin of our elder years, the body's largest organ requires care and awareness at every stage. Skincare, often perceived as a complex regimen, begins with basic yet powerful steps. In this chapter, we will explore fundamental skincare practices including Cleansing, Exfoliation, Gentle Application, Moisturizing, Sun Protection, Understanding Skin Types, Establishing a Routine, and Hygienic Practices.

Cleansing: The Cornerstone of Skincare

Cleansing is the bedrock upon which a solid skincare routine is built. It involves the removal of dirt, oil, and other environmental pollutants that accumulate on the skin's surface and can contribute to irritations and breakouts. A gentle cleanser, suited to your skin type, used morning and evening, prepares the skin to absorb other products effectively. This simple act, when performed consistently, maintains the skin's clarity and prevents the build-up of impurities that can lead to skin issues.

Exfoliation: Revealing Radiance

Exfoliation refers to the process of sloughing off dead skin cells from the surface of the skin. This reveals the fresh, new cells beneath and promotes a radiant and clear complexion. There are various methods of exfoliation, from physical scrubs to chemical exfoliants. However, the key is moderation; over-exfoliation can strip the skin of its natural oils and disrupt the protective barrier, leading to sensitivity. Typically, exfoliating 1-2 times a week is recommended, though this may vary depending on skin type and sensitivity.

Gentle Application: The Art of Touch

The manner in which we apply products can affect their efficacy and our skin's health. Gentle application ensures that the skin is not pulled or unduly stressed, which can lead to fine lines and sagging over time. Using the soft pads of the fingers, products should be smoothed over the skin in a light, outward motion, allowing for a massage-like effect that promotes circulation without causing damage or irritation.

Moisturizing: Maintaining Skin's Hydration

Next in our skincare symphony is moisturizing. Regardless of your skin type, moisturizing plays a vital role in hydrating and repairing the skin. It works to lock in the moisture and to fortify the skin's natural defense system. Even oily skin benefits from a lightweight, non-comedogenic moisturizer to maintain balance. The act of moisturizing not only plumps the skin but also creates a protective layer against environmental factors.

Sun Protection: A Daily Defense

Often underestimated, sun protection is an absolute non-negotiable in any skincare routine. The sun's ultraviolet rays can cause a myriad of skin issues, from premature aging to serious health conditions like skin cancer. Applying a broad-spectrum sunscreen with at least SPF 30, even on cloudy days, safeguards the skin. It's also important to reapply sunscreen every two hours when exposed to sunlight for prolonged periods.

Understanding Skin Types: The Blueprint of Care

Comprehending your skin type is foundational to selecting the right products and establishing an effective skincare regimen. The common skin types include normal, dry, oily, combination, and sensitive. Each has unique needs and responds differently to various ingredients and formulations. Understanding your skin type allows for a tailored approach to skincare, which in turn yields the best results.

Establishing a Routine: The Rhythm of Results

Consistency is key; establishing a skincare routine and sticking to it is critical for achieving and maintaining skin health. Morning and evening rituals may differ slightly; for example, in the morning, focus on protection against environmental factors, while in the evening, concentrate on repair and hydration. Patience and perseverance in a regular routine are often the most significant contributors to skin improvement.

Hygienic Practices: The Silent Guardians

Lastly, hygienic practices are frequently overlooked but are crucial for skin health. Regularly changing pillowcases, washing makeup brushes and sponges, and avoiding the temptation to touch one's face excessively can prevent bacterial transfer and mitigate breakouts. In the same vein, products should be stored properly and replaced as per their expiration dates to avoid skin irritation or infections.

To conclude, basic skincare is an ode to the dermatological canvas we all bear. It is both a practice in self-care and a testament to healthful living. While the spectrum of skincare is broad, understanding and adopting these foundational principles will set anyone on a path to a clearer, healthier, and more radiant complexion.

5

Hormones and Their Impact on Skin

Introduction to Hormonal Influence on Skin

The skin, being the largest organ of the body, is not just a barrier between the internal organs and the external environment—it's also a canvas marked by the ebb and flow of the hormones within our bodies. Hormones act as messengers that can alter the behavior of cells, and with them, the appearance and well-being of our skin. Understanding the interplay between hormones and skin is vital for effective skincare practices.

The Endocrine System and the Skin

To comprehend the hormonal influence on skin, it's essential to briefly explore the endocrine system. This network of glands secretes hormones directly into the circulatory system, regulating numerous body functions including growth, metabolism, and mood. The skin has receptors for various hormones which means fluctuations in these biochemicals can manifest in skin changes such as oil production, elasticity, and regeneration.

Acne and Hormones

The Connection Between Hormones and Sebum Production

Acne is one of the most visible effects of hormones on the skin. Sebaceous glands, which produce oil, or sebum, are stimulated by androgens such as testosterone. While necessary for skin lubrication, overproduction due to hormonal surges (such as during puberty) can lead to clogged pores and breakouts.

Treating Hormonal Acne

Treatment options often include topical retinoids or antimicrobials, oral contraceptives (in women), or medications like spironolactone that reduce androgen activity. Each of these treatments targets the hormonal pathways that exacerbate acne, illustrating the critical role hormones play in skin health.

Menstrual Cycle Effects on Skin

Phases of the Menstrual Cycle and Skin

Throughout the menstrual cycle, fluctuations in estrogen and progesterone levels have visible effects on the skin. During ovulation, increased estrogen may contribute to a clearer, glowy appearance. In contrast, the luteal phase can trigger oiliness, puffiness, and the dreaded premenstrual breakout.

Skincare Adjustments Throughout the Cycle

Recognizing these patterns allows for a tailored skincare approach—perhaps lighter, non-comedogenic products during the oily phase and more hydrating, soothing components when dryness ensues.

Hormonal Imbalances and Skin Manifestations

Beyond routine fluctuations, hormonal imbalances can lead to conditions like hirsutism, hyperpigmentation, or atypical acne. Conditions like polycystic ovary syndrome (PCOS) can lead to excessive androgens and subsequently more severe acne, increased facial hair, and skin tags.

Diagnostics and Skin-focused Treatments

Diagnostics for suspected hormone-related skin issues include blood tests and possibly imaging. Treatments may involve lifestyle changes, medication to correct hormonal imbalances, and topical treatments to address the skin concerns directly.

Hormone Replacement Therapy and Skin Health

The Role of HRT in Skincare for Menopausal Women

As women enter menopause, reduced estrogen levels can lead to dryness, loss of elasticity, and thinning of the skin. Hormone replacement therapy (HRT) often helps mitigate these effects by supplementing the body's hormone levels, thereby restoring some normalcy to the skin's appearance.

The Benefits and Risks of HRT

While HRT can have rejuvenating effects on menopausal skin, it's not without risks, including an increased risk of certain cancers and cardiovascular issues. Consequently, the decision to use HRT should be made on an individual basis, weighing all potential benefits and risks.

The relationship between hormones and skin is complex and profoundly influential to one's skin health. Acne, menstrual cycle effects, and other hormonal imbalances play pivotal roles in the integrity and appearance of our skin. Advancements in understanding hormonal pathways and their connection to skin have led to targeted treatments in acne, aging, and other dermatological conditions.

In summary, a holistic approach that takes hormonal influences into account can lead to a more comprehensive and effective skincare regimen. Hormones will continue to challenge our skin throughout various stages of life, but with knowledge and appropriate care, we can respond in kind to maintain the health and vitality of our largest organ.

Next in this series, we will examine the nutritional aspects of skincare and how diet can affect hormonal balance and, consequently, skin health.

6

The Gut-Skin Connection: Nourishing Beauty from Within

The Gut-Skin Axis: Understanding the Link

In the complex and interconnected systems of the human body, perhaps one of the most surprising links is that between our gut and our skin. Recent dermatological research has provided compelling evidence supporting the gut-skin axis—a bidirectional relationship demonstrating that our digestive health directly impacts our skin's condition.

The gut-skin connection posits that an imbalance in our digestive system, particularly within our gut microbiota, can manifest externally as a range of skin issues. These can vary from acne and eczema to premature aging. This relationship is founded on the understanding that the gut communicates with the skin through multiple pathways, including immune system responses, nutrient absorption, and stress signaling.

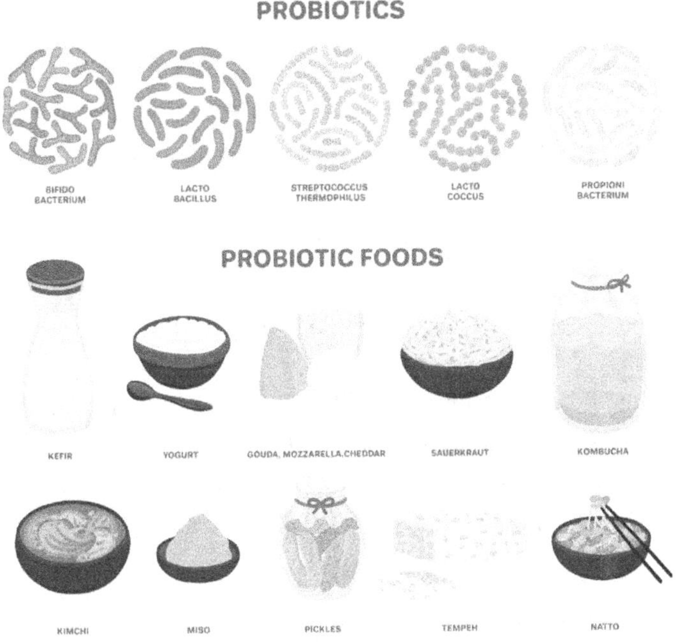

Inflammation: The Common Culprit Behind Skin Issues

Central to the gut-skin dynamic is the role of inflammation. Inflammation is the body's natural response to injury or infection, but when it becomes chronic, it can wreak havoc on both the intestinal lining and the skin barrier. In conditions like inflammatory bowel disease (IBD), we often see concurrent dermatological disorders that underscore this connection.

The skin, being an immune-responsive organ, reflects internal imbalances. Therefore, a gut inflamed by food sensitivities, allergies, or infections can lead to inflamed skin manifesting as rosacea, acne, or other inflammatory skin conditions.

The Gut Microbiome: A Delicate Ecosystem Impacting Skin Health

Our gut microbiome consists of trillions of bacteria, both helpful and harmful. This delicate ecosystem plays a critical role in digestion, immune function, and even influences our mood. When this balance tips, it can lead to a condition known as "dysbiosis," with potential effects on skin health indicating that our microbiota composition is crucial for maintaining clear, healthy skin.

Abundant and diverse beneficial bacteria aid in reducing the systemic presence of pathogens and toxins, which, in turn, curbs the incidence of skin flare-ups. Hence, maintaining a healthy gut microbiome becomes paramount in caring for our skin indirectly.

Dietary Impact: You Are What You Digest

Our diet significantly impacts our gut health, and by extension, our skin's clarity and luminosity. Diets high in processed foods, sugar, and unhealthy fats can disrupt our gut microbiota and promote the growth of bacteria linked to skin conditions like acne. Conversely, a diet rich in fiber, vitamins, antioxidants, and minerals supports a robust microbiome. This dietary approach also lessens oxidative stress and inflammation—both of which can prematurely age skin.

Foods such as omega-3-rich salmon, colorful fruits and vegetables, and fermented items can bolster our gut health, leading to a radiant complexion. The message is clear: what we put into our bodies is reflected on the outside.

Probiotics and Skincare: Allies in Achieving Optimal Skin Health

Probiotics are beneficial bacteria that, when ingested or applied topically, can enhance the bacterial profile of our gut and skin. In terms of ingestion, probiotic supplements or probiotic-rich foods such as kefir, sauerkraut, and yogurt can help restore gut health, which may in turn alleviate certain skin concerns.

In skincare, topical probiotics can act on the skin's surface to protect against harmful bacteria, reduce inflammation, and strengthen the skin's barrier function. By incorporating probiotics in both diet and skincare routines, we can support our skin's health from both the inside and out.

When we talk about skin health, the discussion is incomplete without acknowledging the powerful influence of our gut health. It is this internal-external connection that opens a pathway to not just treating but truly understanding an array of skin conditions and diseases. As such, integrating a gut-conscious perspective into skincare regimens and overall wellness habits may be one of the most holistic approaches we can adopt in our quest for true and lasting beauty.

To manifest optimal skin health, we must look beyond the surface and consider the health and balance of our internal systems—starting with the gut. It's clear that the most luminous beauty emerges from a well-nourished foundation—a testament to the profound connection between what we consume and the outward expression of our health. The gut-skin connection is not just about beauty; it's about fostering harmonious health that radiates from the inside out.

7

Navigating Common Skin Concerns

I n the landscape of skin health, it is normal to traverse a variety of terrains. Each individual's skin narrates the unique story of their genetics, lifestyle, and environmental interactions. Within these chapters of life, common skin concerns such as acne, eczema, hyperpigmentation, rosacea, and aging emerge as recurring themes. Understanding these conditions is the first step on the journey to healthier skin.

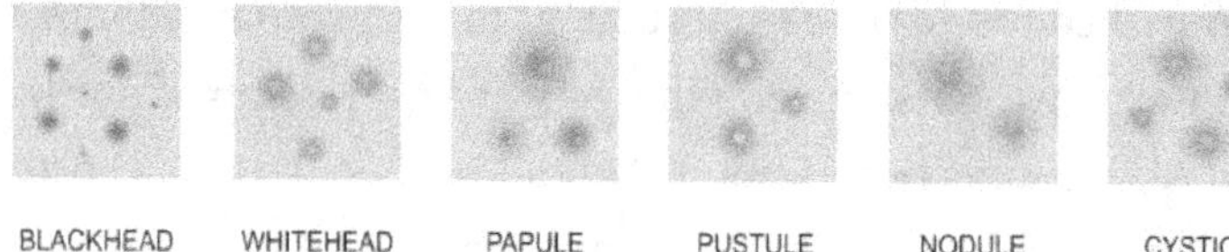

Acne: The Uninvited Guest

Acne is like an uninvited guest that can appear at the doorstep of our skin at any age. Primarily driven by hormonal changes, genetics, stress, and sometimes dietary factors, acne manifests as pimples, blackheads, and painful cysts.

Myth-Busting and Management

Contrary to popular belief, acne isn't just a teenage plight. Many adults experience adult-onset acne, which warrants a different approach to care. Over-the-counter topical treatments containing benzoyl peroxide and salicylic acid can be effective. However, for persistent cases, dermatologists may prescribe antibiotics, retinoids, or hormonal treatments.

Daily Rituals for Prevention:

Regular cleansing to remove excess oil and dirt.

Non-comedogenic makeup and skincare products that won't clog pores.

Adequate hydration and a balanced diet, low in sugar and dairy, may help.

Eczema: More Than Just Dry Skin

Eczema is characterized by red, inflamed, itchy patches on the skin. Often occurring in folds of skin, this condition speaks to an underlying hypersensitivity, which certain irritants or allergens can trigger.

Holistic Approach to Soothe

There is no one-size-fits-all when it comes to managing eczema, but keeping skin well-moisturized is key.

Eczema-friendly Practices:

Use gentle, fragrance-free cleansers and heavy emollients.
   Avoid triggers such as harsh detergents, fabrics like wool, and rapid temperature changes.
   Consider an elimination diet to identify potential food triggers, in consultation with a healthcare provider.

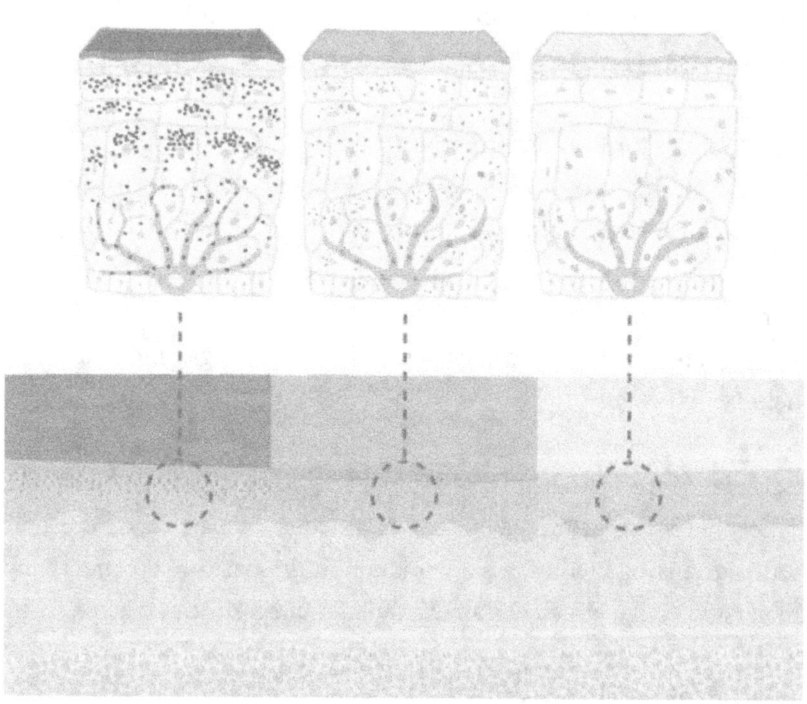

Hyperpigmentation: When Skin Holds onto Memories

Hyperpigmentation appears as darkened patches or spots on the skin, caused by an excess production of melanin, often as a response to factors such as sun exposure, inflammation, or hormonal changes.

Fade and Protect

Treating hyperpigmentation involves a dual approach: fading existing dark spots and preventing further pigmentation.

Skincare Allies:

Ingredients such as vitamin C, kojic acid, and hydroquinone work to fade dark spots.

Sun protection with a broad-spectrum SPF of at least 30 is crucial every day, not just when it's sunny.

A consistent, gentle skincare regimen helps to avoid inflammation, which can trigger further pigmentation.

Rosacea: The Blushing Story

Rosacea presents a narrative of flushing, persistent redness, and sometimes pimple-like bumps, usually on the face. The triggers of rosacea can range from temperature changes to spicy foods.

Mitigating Flare-Ups

Managing rosacea is often about recognizing and avoiding triggers while nurturing the skin with gentle care.

Rosacea Care Commandments:

Use mild skincare products and adopt a gentle cleansing routine.

Protect against sun exposure with physical sunblocks containing zinc oxide or titanium dioxide.

Consult with a dermatologist for treatments such as topical metronidazole, azelaic acid, or oral medications.

Aging-related Concerns: Embracing the Journey

As time writes its chapters on our skin, we may notice the development of wrinkles, loss of elasticity, and changes in texture. Aging is a natural process, but skin aging can be accelerated by lifestyle factors and environmental damage.

Age Gracefully with Care

Embracing aging doesn't mean neglecting skin care. It's about focusing on skin health and prevention.

Youthful Strategies:

Retinoids can assist in cell turnover and collagen production.

Antioxidants like vitamin E and green tea extract help fight free radical damage.

Hydration through products containing hyaluronic acid can plump the skin and reduce the appearance of fine lines.

In conclusion, navigating through common skin concerns requires patience, knowledge, and a personalized approach. While this chapter provides guidance, every skin story is different and may require professional advice. Remember, the journey to healthy skin is ongoing, and embracing it with care will make all the difference.

8

Crafting Effective Skincare Regimens

In this chapter, we will delve into the art of crafting skincare regimens tailored to individual needs. Skincare is a personal journey, and an effective regimen should take into account daily maintenance, skin type, targeted treatments, as well as the differences between morning and evening routines and seasonal adjustments.

Daily Skincare Routine

The foundation of any effective skincare regimen lies in establishing a daily routine. This not only ensures consistency but also allows for a holistic approach to skincare. A basic daily routine includes cleansing, toning, moisturizing, and sun protection. Cleansing helps to remove impurities from the skin, toning rebalances the skin's pH levels, moisturizing provides essential hydration, and sun protection shields the skin from harmful UV rays.

Tailoring to Skin Type

Understanding one's skin type is crucial in creating an effective skincare regimen. Whether your skin is dry, oily, combination, or sensitive, tailoring products to your specific needs can make a significant difference in achieving healthy and radiant skin. For example, those with dry skin may benefit from richer, more emollient moisturizers, while individuals with oily skin may require lighter, oil-free products.

Targeted Treatments

In addition to a basic routine, targeted treatments can address specific skincare concerns such as acne, hyperpigmentation, or aging. Incorporating serums, masks, and specialized treatments into a skincare regimen can help to target and treat these issues effectively. For example, a vitamin C serum can help to brighten and even out the skin tone, while a retinol treatment can diminish fine lines and wrinkles.

Morning vs. Evening Routines

The skin's needs vary throughout the day, necessitating different approaches to morning and evening skincare routines. Morning routines should focus on protection and preparation for the day ahead, including cleansing, moisturizing, and applying SPF. Evening routines, on the other hand, often involve deeper cleansing to remove makeup and impurities, followed by treatments and richer moisturizers to repair and rejuvenate the skin overnight.

Seasonal Adjustments

Skincare regimens should not remain static throughout the year. Seasonal changes in weather, humidity, and temperature can affect the skin, necessitating adjustments to ensure optimal care. For instance, in colder months, a heavier moisturizer may be necessary to combat dryness, while in warmer weather, lighter formulations and increased sun protection are essential.

Crafting an effective skincare regimen is a dynamic process that requires attention to detail, flexibility, and an understanding of individual skin needs. By incorporating daily routines, tailoring products to skin type, targeting specific concerns, adjusting for morning and evening differences, and accommodating seasonal changes, one can achieve a personalized and effective skincare regimen that promotes healthy, glowing skin.

9

Crafting Your Personalized Skincare Routine

When it comes to skincare, there is no one-size-fits-all approach. Each person's skin is unique, and therefore requires a personalized skincare routine. In this chapter, we will discuss how to craft a routine that is tailored to your specific needs and concerns.

Personal Assessment

The first step in crafting your personalized skincare routine is to assess your skin type and specific concerns. Are you dealing with oily skin, dry skin, or a combination of both? Do you struggle with acne, fine lines, or dark spots? Understanding your skin's unique needs will help you choose the right products and treatments.

Product Selection

Once you have assessed your skin, it's time to select the right products for your routine. This may include a gentle cleanser, moisturizer, sunscreen, and targeted treatments such as serums or exfoliants. It's important to choose products that are suited to your skin type and concerns, and to avoid ingredients that may trigger irritation or allergies.

Incorporating Actives

Many skincare enthusiasts choose to incorporate active ingredients into their routine, such as retinoids, vitamin C, or alpha hydroxy acids. These ingredients can target specific concerns like wrinkles, hyperpigmentation, or dullness. When introducing actives into your routine, it's important to start slowly and monitor how your skin responds.

Patch Testing

Before fully incorporating a new product into your routine, it's crucial to conduct a patch test. This involves applying a small amount of the product to a discrete area of your skin, such as behind the ear, and monitoring for any adverse reactions. Patch testing can help you avoid potential allergic reactions or irritation.

Adapting Over Time

As your skin changes with age, seasons, and lifestyle factors, your skincare routine may need to adapt as well. It's important to periodically reassess your skin's needs and make adjustments to your routine as necessary. This could mean swapping out products, adjusting the frequency of certain treatments, or incorporating new products that address evolving concerns.

Crafting a personalized skincare routine is an ongoing process that requires attention, patience, and a willingness to adapt. By taking the time to assess your skin, select the right products, and monitor how your skin responds, you can create a skincare routine that is tailored to your individual needs and helps you achieve your skincare goals.

10

Embracing Anti-Aging Treatments for Radiant Skin

In our quest for timeless beauty, it's essential to understand the key components of effective anti-aging skincare. From retinoids to professional treatments, this chapter will delve into the world of anti-aging and how to embrace treatments that promote youthful, glowing skin.

Retinoids and Retinol:

One of the most potent weapons in the fight against aging is retinoids and retinol. These vitamin A derivatives help to stimulate collagen production, reduce the appearance of fine lines and wrinkles, and improve skin texture. When incorporating retinoids into your skincare routine, it's crucial to start slowly and gradually increase usage to avoid irritation. Additionally, it's essential to use sunscreen daily as retinoids can make the skin more sensitive to the sun.

Moisturization:

Proper moisturization is a fundamental aspect of any anti-aging skincare regimen. As we age, the skin's natural moisture barrier weakens, leading to dryness and an increased appearance of fine lines. Choosing a moisturizer with hydrating ingredients such as hyaluronic acid and glycerin can help replenish the skin's moisture levels, leaving it plump and supple.

Sun Protection:

Sun damage is one of the primary causes of premature aging. Incorporating broad-spectrum sunscreen into your daily routine is crucial for preventing photoaging, hyperpigmentation, and the breakdown of collagen. Look for a sunscreen with an SPF of 30 or higher and reapply every two hours, especially when spending prolonged periods outdoors.

Antioxidants:

Antioxidants play a pivotal role in neutralizing free radicals, which can cause oxidative stress and accelerate the aging process. Including antioxidant-rich products in your skincare routine, such as vitamin C serums and green tea extracts, can help protect the skin from environmental aggressors and promote a more youthful complexion.

Professional Treatments:

In addition to at-home skincare, professional treatments can provide targeted solutions for addressing signs of aging. Options such as chemical peels, microdermabrasion, and laser therapy can help to reduce the appearance of fine lines, stimulate collagen production, and improve overall skin tone and texture. Consulting with a dermatologist or licensed skincare professional can help determine the most suitable professional treatments for your specific skincare concerns.

In conclusion, embracing anti-aging treatments is a proactive approach to maintaining healthy, radiant skin. By incorporating retinoids and retinol, prioritizing moisturization, practicing diligent sun protection, harnessing the power of antioxidants, and considering professional treatments, you can embark on a journey towards gracefully aging skin that radiates vitality and youthfulness.

11

Maximizing Your Skincare Routine with the Power of Skincare Tools

Skincare tools have become essential companions in the quest for healthy, radiant skin. From cleansing brushes to facial rollers, these tools offer a myriad of benefits that complement and elevate traditional skincare practices. In this chapter, we explore how to harness the power of skincare tools to enhance your skincare regimen and achieve optimal results.

Cleansing Brushes:

Cleansing brushes have revolutionized the way we cleanse our skin. These devices, equipped with gentle bristles, provide a thorough and deep cleanse, effectively removing dirt, makeup, and impurities from the skin's surface. When using a cleansing brush, it's important to choose one that suits your skin type and sensitivity. Incorporating a cleansing brush into your routine can help unclog pores, promote better absorption of skincare products, and leave the skin feeling fresh and revitalized.

Facial Rollers:

Facial rollers, often crafted from jade or rose quartz, have gained popularity for their rejuvenating and soothing properties. These handheld tools, typically featuring dual ends, are used to massage the skin, reduce puffiness, and enhance the penetration of serums and moisturizers. When used in conjunction with skincare products, facial rollers can promote lymphatic drainage, improve circulation, and impart a radiant, lifted appearance to the skin.

LED Light Therapy Devices:

LED light therapy devices utilize various wavelengths of light to address an array of skincare concerns, including acne, inflammation, and signs of aging. By emitting specific wavelengths, these devices stimulate cellular activity, promote collagen production, and help to alleviate skin conditions. Incorporating LED light therapy into your skincare routine can have transformative effects, offering targeted solutions for achieving clear, youthful, and radiant skin.

Microcurrent Devices:

Microcurrent devices have garnered attention for their ability to stimulate facial muscles, improve tone, and enhance overall firmness. Through gentle electrical currents, these handheld devices encourage muscle re-education and lift, leading to a more contoured and sculpted appearance. When used consistently, microcurrent devices can contribute to a more youthful complexion, improving the skin's elasticity and reducing the visibility of fine lines and wrinkles.

Facial Cleansing Devices:

Facial cleansing devices, such as sonic brushes and silicone cleansing pads, provide an effective and thorough method of cleansing the skin. These devices utilize technology to deeply cleanse and exfoliate the skin, promoting a clearer, smoother complexion. When incorporated into your skincare routine, facial cleansing devices can help remove impurities, minimize the appearance of pores, and maintain the skin's overall health and luminosity.

In summary, harnessing the power of skincare tools can be a transformative addition to your skincare regimen. Whether incorporating cleansing brushes, facial rollers, LED light therapy devices, microcurrent devices, or facial cleansing devices, these tools offer diverse benefits that cater to individual skincare needs. By integrating skincare tools into your routine, you can elevate your skincare experience, achieve optimal results, and bask in the glow of radiant, healthy skin.

12

Skincare Tips for Men: Navigating a Healthy Routine

Men's skincare routines have historically been seen as simplistic, but in recent years, the importance of comprehensive skincare has gained momentum. Navigating a healthy skincare routine as a man involves understanding the unique needs of your skin, simplifying a routine that works for you, and addressing specific concerns. In this chapter, we will explore the essentials of skincare for men, including sun protection, shaving tips, choosing men-friendly products, and how to address specific skincare concerns.

Simplified Routine

For many men, the idea of a detailed skincare routine may seem overwhelming. However, a simplified routine is not only manageable but also highly effective. A basic skincare routine for men should include cleansing, moisturizing, and sun protection. By keeping these steps simple and consistent, men can maintain healthy and vibrant skin without investing excessive time or effort.

Sun Protection

One of the most crucial aspects of skincare for men is sun protection. Even though men's skin may be thicker and have more collagen than women's, it is still susceptible to sun damage. Incorporating a broad-spectrum sunscreen into your daily routine, especially if you spend a significant amount of time outdoors, can prevent premature aging, sunburn, and reduce the risk of skin cancer.

Shaving Tips

Shaving can be a source of irritation for many men, leading to razor burn, ingrown hairs, and sensitivity. To minimize these issues, it's essential to prepare the skin with warm water and a gentle cleanser before shaving. Always use a sharp, clean razor and consider using a shaving cream designed for sensitive skin. After shaving, apply a soothing aftershave lotion to calm the skin and prevent irritation.

Choosing Men-Friendly Products

When selecting skincare products, it's important to choose those tailored specifically for men's skin. Men often have oilier and thicker skin, so products designed to address these concerns can be beneficial. Look for products with lightweight, non-greasy formulations and ingredients such as salicylic acid or witch hazel to control oil and prevent breakouts.

Skincare for Specific Concerns

Men may also have specific skincare concerns, such as acne, sensitivity, or signs of aging. Tailoring your skincare routine to address these concerns is essential for maintaining healthy, balanced skin. For example, using a gentle cleanser and non-comedogenic moisturizer can help manage acne-prone skin, while incorporating a retinol-based product can address signs of aging.

In conclusion, navigating a healthy skincare routine as a man involves embracing a simplified yet effective regimen. By prioritizing sun protection, implementing shaving tips, choosing men-friendly products, and addressing specific skincare concerns, men can achieve optimal skin health and appearance. Remember, skincare is not just a luxury; it's an essential part of overall health and well-being.

13

Mastering Skincare on the Go: Essential Travel Tips

When it comes to travel, maintaining a proper skincare routine can be challenging. Whether you are a seasoned traveler or a frequent flyer, the ability to maintain healthy, glowing skin while on the go is essential. Thankfully, with the right products and techniques, you can master skincare on the go without sacrificing your skin's health.

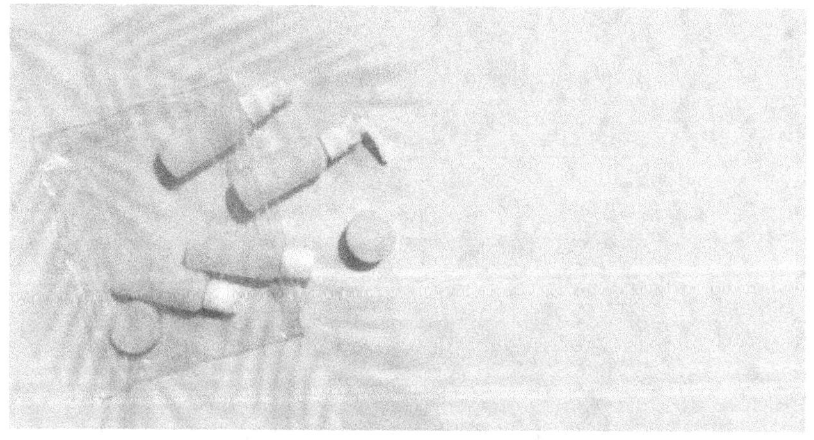

Lightweight Products for Portability

When traveling, it's important to streamline your skincare routine by opting for lightweight products that are easy to carry. Look for serums, moisturizers, and cleansers that come in travel-sized containers to minimize weight and maximize space in your luggage. Lightweight, non-greasy formulas are perfect for on-the-go skincare, as they absorb quickly and won't weigh you down during your travels.

Efficient Multi-Tasking Products

With limited space in your suitcase, multitasking skincare products can be a game-changer. Consider using a versatile tinted moisturizer with SPF, which provides hydration, sun protection, and a touch of color in one step. Additionally, there are multi-purpose balms that can be used for moisturizing lips, soothing dry patches, and taming unruly eyebrows. By packing efficient multi-tasking products, you can simplify your skincare routine while on the go.

Adaptation to Climate

Travel often means exposure to different climates and environmental conditions. It's essential to adapt your skincare routine to accommodate these changes. If you're heading to a dry climate, focus on hydrating products such as hyaluronic acid serums and rich moisturizers. For humid destinations, opt for lightweight, oil-free products that won't clog your pores. By understanding the impact of climate on your skin, you can ensure that your skincare routine remains effective no matter where you are in the world.

Hydration and Protection

Maintaining proper hydration and sun protection is crucial, whether you're on a beach vacation or exploring a bustling city. Invest in a hydrating facial mist to keep your skin refreshed and moisturized throughout the day. Additionally, never forget the importance of sunscreen. Choose a broad-spectrum SPF that suits your skin type and apply it religiously, especially when spending time outdoors. Hydration and protection are non-negotiable components of any travel skincare routine.

Travel-Friendly Packaging

When selecting skincare products for travel, consider the packaging. Opt for products that come in travel-friendly containers, such as pump bottles, squeezy tubes, or solid sticks. These types of packaging are less likely to leak or spill in your luggage, making them ideal for hassle-free travel. Look for brands that offer refillable travel containers or sample sizes of their products, further maximizing convenience and minimizing bulk.

In conclusion, mastering skincare on the go is all about strategic product selection and adaptability. By choosing lightweight, multitasking products, adapting to climate changes, prioritizing hydration and protection, and favoring travel-friendly packaging, you can maintain glowing, healthy skin no matter where your travels take you. With these essential travel tips, your skincare routine can seamlessly integrate into your adventures, ensuring that you look and feel your best while exploring the world.

14

Conclusion

Throughout *The Skincare Lab*, we have explored the diverse facets of skincare, delving into the intricacies of skincare routines, product selection, and the importance of holistic skincare practices. From understanding skin types and identifying personalized routines to exploring the benefits of specific ingredients and mastering skincare on the go, each chapter has been an essential piece of the puzzle in achieving radiant and healthy skin.

We have emphasized the significance of tailored skincare approaches, acknowledging that each individual's skin is unique and deserves its own personalized regimen. By unraveling the complexities of skincare, we have equipped you with the knowledge and tools necessary to curate a skincare routine that aligns with your skin's specific needs and preferences.

Furthermore, we have highlighted the transformative power of key skincare components, emphasizing the roles of cleansers, serums, moisturizers, and treatments in nurturing and maintaining skin health. By understanding the influence of ingredients and their effects on the skin, you are empowered to make informed decisions when selecting products that harmonize with your skin's requirements.

In this concluding chapter, we have unraveled the art of mastering skincare on the go, recognizing the challenges of maintaining a skincare regimen while traveling and providing invaluable tips to circumvent these challenges. Through the incorporation of lightweight products, efficient multitasking elements, climate adaptation, hydration and protection strategies, and travel-friendly packaging, we have established a roadmap for seamless skincare maintenance during your adventures.

Collectively, our exploration of skincare has emphasized the fusion of knowledge, intentionality, and adaptability in achieving skincare mastery. By embracing the multifaceted approach to skincare and adopting practices that honor your skin's unique composition, you are embarking on a journey of self-care and nurturing that transcends superficial beauty—an odyssey that celebrates the embodiment of radiant, healthy skin as a reflection of inner vitality and well-being.

As you conclude this enlightening journey through the world of skincare, remember that the secrets to skincare mastery lie within your grasp. Armed with comprehensive insights and a deepened understanding of effective skincare practices, you are well-equipped to embark on a lifelong expedition of skincare enrichment, empowerment, and luminosity.

Now, as our exploration of skincare draws to a close, we encourage readers to reflect on their experiences with this book. We invite you to leave a review, sharing your thoughts, insights, and the ways in which this content has impacted your approach to skincare. Your feedback will help inform and inspire others on their own skincare odyssey. Thank you for joining us on this transformative journey.

If you found this book helpful, I'd be very appreciative if you left a favorable review for this book on amazon!